K9
Tactical
First Aid

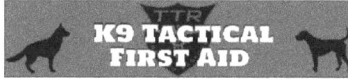

Laura J. Kendall

Basic Emergency Treatment for a Severe Arterial Bleed

If safe to do so then call out for help!

Apply medical gloves or something to protect yourself from blood.

↓

Perform an **RTA MARCH** to find life threatening bleeding.

↓

Arterial Bleed? - YES!

Begin by applying **Direct Pressure** to the bleeding site.

↓

Bleeding does not stop with direct pressure!

↓

Pack the wound using hemostatic or regular gauze & apply a pressure dressing. Continue holding direct pressure on the wound.

↓

Extremity wound – consider application of an appropriate tourniquet.

Keep the animal lying down & warm. Reassure them in a calm voice.

Unresponsive - place in the recovery position. Monitor & continue controlling the bleeding site. **Do not pack the head, chest, abdomen or back!**

K9 CPR Steps

Check for unresponsiveness – approach from the side or back calling their name & making noise.

Unresponsive – Yes!

Check for breathing – open the airway by aligning the pet's head/neck – look, listen and feel for breathing - not breathing – pull out tongue slightly – close mouth and seal your mouth over the dog's nose and blow into the dog's nose giving two breaths.

Breaths goes in – Yes - Check for pulse – no pulse – start chest compressions.

Do 30 compressions – 2 breaths – do for 2 minutes (5 times of 30-2) and recheck for pulse and breathing.

How fast to compress -Rate: 100-120 per minute and allow full chest recoil (keep hands on chest) Think of the song – Staying Alive.

Rescue breathing –Dog has a pulse, but is not breathing. Initiate mouth to snout breaths- **give one breath approximately every 3 – 6 seconds.**

Hand Placement

Medium - Large dog – Place dog on their side. Compress with hands placed directly behind dog's front leg/armpit. This is the area closest to the dog's heart.

Puppy – small dog – Perform CPR by cupping your hand. One hand underneath dog and other hand over chest. Use top hand to compress.

Barrel Chested Dog – Place on back and compress in center of dog's chest.

Important Numbers

Emergency Services – call 911 or your country specific emergency number if you are in danger or the animal is in danger.

Local Police Department Non- Emergent Number:

Local Fire Department Non – Emergent Number:

Regular Vet Phone:

1. Emergency 24-hour vet
Phone:
Address:

2. Emergency 24-hour vet
Phone:
Address:

Pet Poison Control Helpline: 855-886-7965
(fee per incident)

Emergency Care Vet Report

Pet's Name:

Age:

Breed:

S – Signs & Symptoms

A- Allergies (medications, food & any others)

M- Current Medications they are taking

P – Past Medical History & Conditions

L – Last Meal or Drink

E- Events : Paint a clear picture for the vet of what happened.

Vital Signs – Pulse Rate: Breathing Rate:

Color of gums:

Treatment you provided for your pet:

Medications you administered:

Did the treatment help?

Pet Insurance:

Content

Welcome

Module 1: SMART – Scene Safety, Muzzle, Assess, Rapidly Treat, Transport.

Module 2: Scene Safety.

Module 3: Muzzling an injured animal.

Module 4: Assessment, vital signs.

Module 5: Rapidly treat life threats, The MARCH Assessment , Direct pressure, Hemostatic gauze, pressure bandages, tourniquets.

Module 6: Impaled objects, fractures, spinal injuries, tail injuries, internal bleeding, bite wounds, foot injuries, shock, bloat.

Module 7: Preparing to give report to the emergency vet using SAMPLE, my go to supplies for your trauma kits.

Conclusion

Resources

Works Cited

Cover Models: K9 Benning, K9 LEO Justin & K9 Anna.

Cover Photo by Joni McKelvey.

Definitions

Immediate Responder: A person who recognizes a bleeding injury and acts to save lives.

EV: Emergency Veterinarian .

GSW: Gunshot Wound.

RTA: Rapid Trauma Assessment.

Tactical Trauma Care: A specific set of action steps utilized to provide immediate treatment of traumatically injured victims.

Triage: The act of sorting victims according to the seriousness of their injuries and from this treatment and transportation decisions are made.

TQ: Tourniquet

Dedication

This book in memory of my heart dogs. To my Yellow Lab, and fur-son, Barky Bear and to The Greyhound Gals and fur-daughters KD Kelsey, Make Me Blush, and Queen of the Nights.

I thank you for your unconditional love and my only wish is that our pets live longer. I miss you all more than words can ever convey.

I also dedicate this to you, my reader, because you are taking the proactive and much needed stance of learning what to do when an animal is injured or ill and how to help save lives using basic bleeding care, pet first aid and equipment.

Having knowledge and action steps to take during a critical incident is key to saving lives.

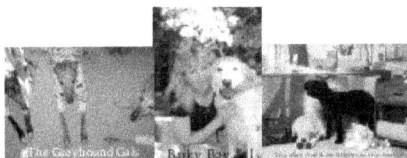

Acknowledgements

I would like to acknowledge the following agencies and sites for their invaluable wealth on assess, treating, stabilizing and transporting an injured pet to an emergency vet. Please take time to go to their websites and read the information as well as watch the videos.

TacMed Solutions - K9 Tourniquet

Deployed Medicine

CoK9CCC Guidelines

CoTCCC Guidelines

Paws N Claws 911 in-person Pet First Aid & CPR class taught by owner Tom Rinelli

Igor Yankin, DVM, DACVECC - online class on hemorrhagic shock in small animals

North American Rescue

Rapid Application Tourniquets

National Safety Council

Thank You!

A huge thank you to my Editor and EMT extraordinaire – Michele Hess. Not only have you helped me on EMS calls, you are making sure this manual looks professional and clean. Thank you my friend!!!

Any spelling or punctuation errors after your editing are purely mine.

Foreword

I've been in the field of EMS since 1981 and a NJ Mobile Intensive Care paramedic since 1986, retiring from the street in 2018. I'm also an animal lover, dog & cat mom and greyhound foster mom.

In my years as an emergency care provider, I've encountered injured animals and assessed them for injury. As a pet mom and foster mom, I've dealt with my yellow lab getting Bloat and surviving because I trusted my gut. I've also dealt with my two greyhounds getting brutally attacked by a dog that broke through the "invisible" fence and horrifically injured them. They required immediate transportation to a vet for surgery and weeks of after-care and medicine. In fact, it was during this time I received my first and only write up as a paramedic for taking time off to care for my dogs! To me, our fur-babies are just as important as the rest of our family and I, personally, did not hesitate to step up and care for mine – no matter what it cost me.

I hope you use this book as a guide and support system should your dog be injured. By knowing simple First Aid, you can step up and be a pet parent hero to your fur-baby, just as I was to mine. Stay safe my friends!

Laura J. Kendall – CEO Train To Respond, LLC

Other books by Laura J. Kendall

The Bleed Control Specialist Manual – Humans

Active Shooter Response & Tactical Trauma Care
Manual

The Rescue Task Force & Tactical Trauma Care
Manual

for EMS, FIRE, and Law Enforcement.

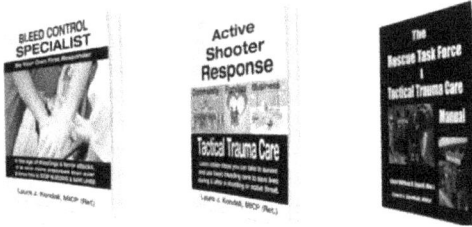

We offer Live Training & Education Courses
Learn more at www.traintorespond.com

Module One

Acronym SMART

S: Is the scene safe for you to enter?

M: Muzzle the dog or restrain the small dog.

A: Assess the animal for life threatening injuries.

R: Rapidly treat the life threats.

T: Transport to the emergency vet/hospital.

Module Two

S

Scene safety requires you to trust your gut as well as approach the injured animal with caution. <u>Your safety always comes first.</u>

Be aware of traffic if the animal has been injured in or near a roadway. Many well-meaning animal rescuers have been killed by vehicles.

Remember, as well, that animals in pain or scared may be unpredictable and aggressive. I always used to say, when working as a paramedic, that if a person bites me (they have) they mean to harm me, but if a dog bites me they are doing it out of fear and to protect themselves. This is why it is important to approach an injured animal slowly, remain calm and avoid direct eye contact.

Also, if you can approach the animal from the side or behind this may be less threatening to them. Speak in a calm and reassuring voice.

While approaching the injured animal observe how they are acting. Do they appear in distress? Are they exhibiting signs of fear and aggression? How do they respond to treats or food you might use to gain trust?

Injured dogs should be muzzled unless a contraindication to muzzling is noted during your assessment. Muzzling a dog or restraining a small dog (using a blanket wrap or other method) is for your safety as well as theirs.

Apply medical gloves to protect yourself against disease.

Module Three
M

Muzzle or restrain the injured animal for your safety and for theirs.

Contraindications to muzzling!!!

1. Do not muzzle an animal that is vomiting!

2. Do not muzzle an animal having trouble breathing!

3. Do not muzzle an animal with mouth injuries!

4. Do not muzzle an animal having an active seizure!

5. Do not muzzle an unconscious animal!

The issues that prevent muzzling have to do with maintaining an open airway and, if required, initiating mouth to snout breathing or CPR.

There are commercial muzzles of all sizes you can purchase or you can makeshift a muzzle using a strip of fabric, belt, or leash.

Small dogs without a large snout can be restrained by wrapping them in a blanket, towel or other item you have available.

If bitten by a dog, you should also seek evaluation by a medical professional for treatment, especially if the rabies status of the animal who bit you is in question.

When muzzling an animal, the goal is to keep their mouth closed enough so they can't bite you, but not so tight it causes injury to them. This is a quick and easy way to muzzle a dog.

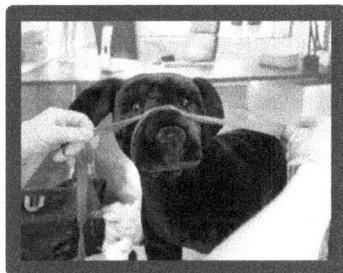

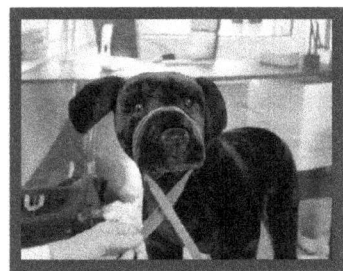

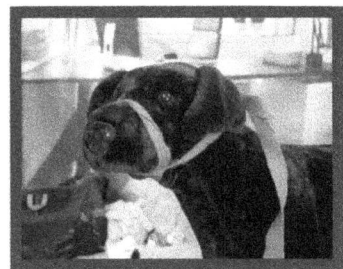

Module Four

A

Rapid Trauma Assessment – RTA

A popular assessment for both people and pets is The MARCH assessment

M – assess for and control Massive bleeding. This is the first priority as it is the quickest killer and one that can be rapidly treated to save lives.

A – assess is their Airway open? If the injured animal is growling, whining or barking this tells you automatically their airway is open. If not then open the airway. (we will cover this in the treatment section of this manual.)

R – assess for Respirations. Are they breathing? Do you see chest rise and fall? Count how many breaths they take in fifteen seconds and multiply by four to get their breaths per minute.

Normal respirations for a dog are between 10 – 30 breaths per minute.

C – assess for a Pulse (Circulation). Do they have a pulse? Is it rapid, weak or absent? Feel the pulse for 15 seconds and multiply the number of beats felt by fifteen. This will give you beats per minute.

Check for a dog's pulse on the inside of their upper back leg – this is where the femoral pulse is located.

Normal baseline heart rates:

Dog over 30 pounds = between 60 – 100 beats per minute.

Dogs under 30 pounds = between 100 – 140 beats per minute.

Puppies = 120 – 160 beats per minute.

All heart rates will depend on how fit the animal is, their age, activity level and medical conditions.

You can also check for perfusion by pressing on their gums. Be careful you do not get bit. Press on the gum and count how many seconds it takes for normal color to return. It should take less than two seconds. You can try this on yourself right now by pressing on your nail bed and counting how many seconds it takes for color to return. As in our pets, it should take humans less than two seconds as well.

Normal gums are pink in color and healthy looking.

Pale gums = shock.

Blue gums = lack of oxygen – cyanosis.

Remember to protect yourself from blood borne diseases as best as possible in these situations.

H –assess for body temp. (Hypothermia) It's important to maintain a normal body temperature. Keep them warm. (We will discuss this further in the treatment section).

Rapid Bleeding Assessment:

A good way of assessing for bleeding and to find all the holes or punctures is to put your open hands close together. Bend the tops of your fingers down and rapidly rake them down the animal's body.

By keeping your hands together with fingers slightly bent you can make sure you don't miss any areas while feeling for puncture wounds.

Cover all areas of the animal's body.

Start at the neck, front & back legs, core (head, chest, belly, back), and tail.

You must check for both entrance and exit wounds, especially if the animal has been shot!

When you find bleeding, immediately begin treatment to stop it! We will cover this in-depth in the next section of this manual.

Remember, if an animal or human suffers injury to an artery, they can bleed out rapidly! Sometimes in under a minute! This is why bleeding is the first thing we check for in an injured animal or human.

Time is our enemy when someone is bleeding. Your assessment should take no more than thirty seconds and bleeding control in sixty seconds or less.

Module Five

R

Rapidly treat all life threats you have found on assessment!

Massive Bleeding

Bleeding

Remember to protect yourself against bloodborne diseases, if possible, by wearing medical gloves or a sealed protective barrier over your skin.

Three types of bleeding:

Capillary Bleeding

Smallest blood vessels that deliver oxygenated blood to the tissues and take back deoxygenated blood to the veins. Capillary bleeding is slow and oozes out. It stops quickly with direct pressure.

Venous Bleeding

Veins carry blood with little to no oxygen in them which explains the dark red color. They are not under pressure and bleed slow and steady.

Deep cuts have the potential to cut open veins.

The best way to stop most cases of venous bleeding is to put direct pressure on the wound. This is when a Pressure Bandage would be applied to help slow and stop the bleeding.

But remember, we are not stopping the pulse in the affected area, so not too tight!

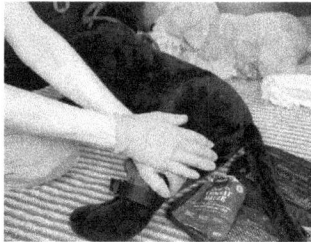

Arterial Bleeding – the deadly killer!

Arteries carry freshly oxygenated blood (which is why arteries have bright red blood in them) from the heart to be distributed to the tissues of the body. Because they carry rich oxygenated blood that must go throughout the body, they are under pressure. This is why arterial bleeds are so deadly.

Arterial bleeding is the least common but the deadliest type of bleeding. In an arterial bleed, the blood **is** bright red and spurts out each time the heart beats. Picture a garden hose on at full blast. This is what a bleed of a major artery looks like. **Literally, the victim will die in 1 - 5 minutes if no first aid is given.**

In most cases of arterial bleeding, direct and extremely firm pressure on the wound is the best way of stopping it.

If direct pressure is not applied, a severe arterial wound can cause you to bleed to death within a few minutes.

Arterial bleeding may be hard to notice right away if the animal has dark fur or if it's a dark environment. You will need to look, do a hands-on assessment and watch for pooling of blood in one spot.

MARCH

March- **Treating massive bleeding in a Canine**

The number one step you can take to stop bleeding is to apply direct pressure.

Direct pressure means to apply pressure by applying your gloved hands and a dressing directly on top of the wound. Push down. This will compress the bleeding vessel against a bone and help the vessel to begin to form a clot.

If you notice bleeding coming through the dressing you have applied – DO NOT REMOVE IT! By removing the dressing, you will dislodge any clots that have begun to form.

Instead, apply more dressings on top of the first one and continue to apply direct pressure.

If direct pressure does not stop bleeding then other measures are called for.

The following information is coming directly from the updated May of 2023 Canine/K9 Tactical Combat Casualty Care Guidelines.

For dogs, if bleeding does not stop with direct pressure, the next step is to pack the wound using hemostatic gauze and apply a pressure dressing.

Although we will cover tourniquet application in pets next, they have drawbacks due to anatomy differences and their ability to stop bleeding in a canine is not as effective as it is in a human.

Hemostatic / Combat Gauze

Hemostatic Gauze is a chemical agent that stops bleeding. There are several different kinds.

Hemostatic Gauze is used in a canine when direct pressure does not stop the hemorrhaging.

➡It is important to be trained in the use of hemostatic gauze and feel confident in your ability to use it properly and when needed.

Types of hemostatic gauze

Quick Clot / Combat Gauze: This is gauze impregnated with Kaolin and helps to activate the patient's own clotting system.

It may not work as well or at all in the absence of the patients clotting factors due to hypothermia, massive blood loss or blood thinner medications.

Celox – Chito Gauze: This is gauze impregnated with chitosan, which is derived from crustaceans.

This has not been shown to cause any allergic reactions to shellfish sensitive patients due to the way it is made.

Celox works in absence of the patient's own clotting factors. It works by absorbing blood/fluid and forming a gel like plug to cover the wound and stop bleeding.

How to use hemostatic gauze.

Step 1: **Tear open Hemostatic Gauze pouch** at the indicated tear notches **and take out the Hemostatic Gauze.**

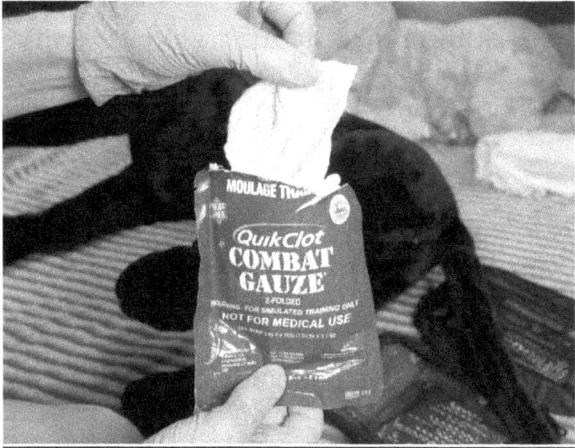

Step 2: Pack the Hemostatic Gauze all the way down into the wound cavity until you make contact with the severed or torn artery.

Human

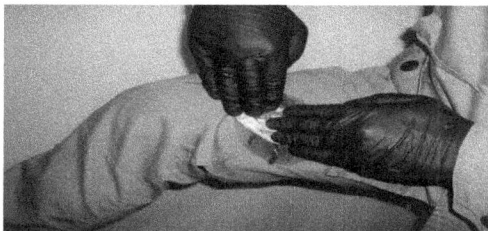

Pet

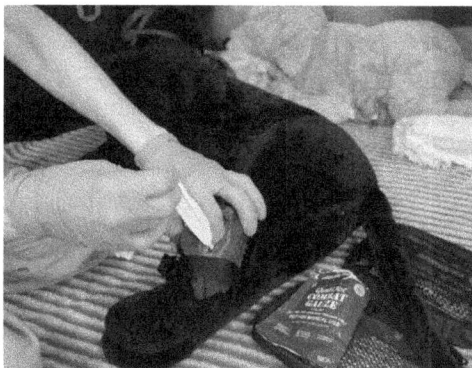

<u>Step 3:</u> Immediately apply direct pressure and hold that for at least <u>5 minutes.</u> If using regular gauze and not hemostatic gauze hold pressure for at least 10 minutes.

Human

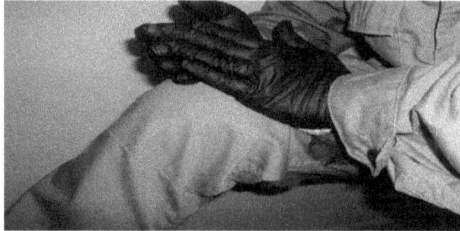

Pet

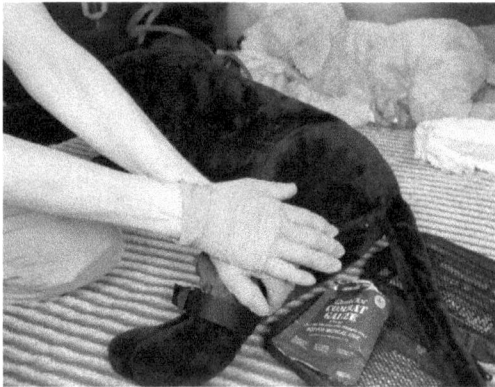

Pressure Bandages

Pressure bandages are used to control venous bleeding that is able to be slowed or stopped using direct pressure.

How to use a pressure bandage:

<u>Deploy Emergency Pressure Bandage with non-stick pad directly over the wound</u>

Human

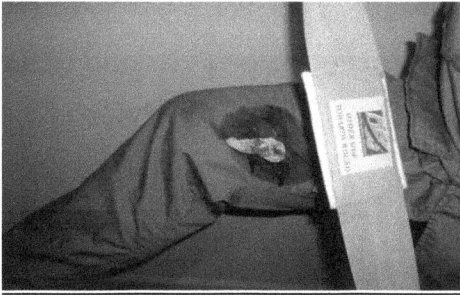

Pet

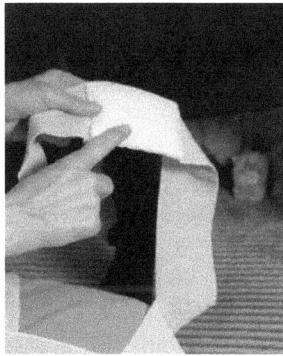

Wrap tightly creating pressure to be forced down onto the wound.

Human

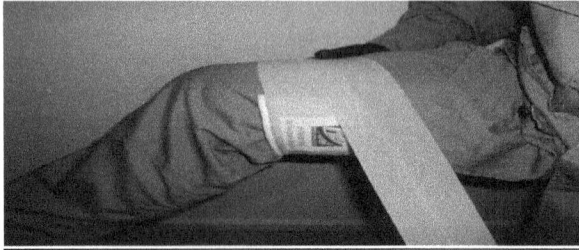

Pet

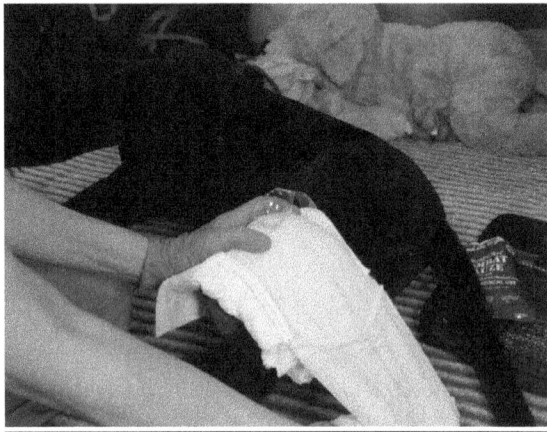

Wrap an inch below the wound and an inch above the wound

Human

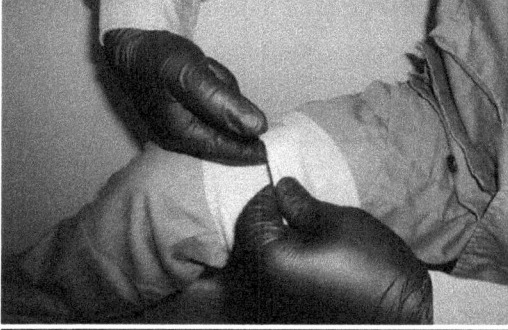

Pet

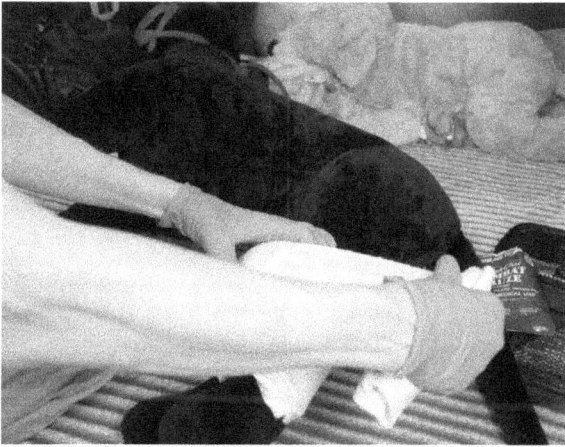

Secure by affixing the end onto the wrap

Human

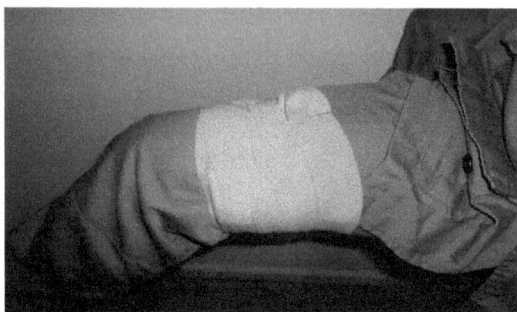

Human Images courtesy of Marc Barry OSS

Pet

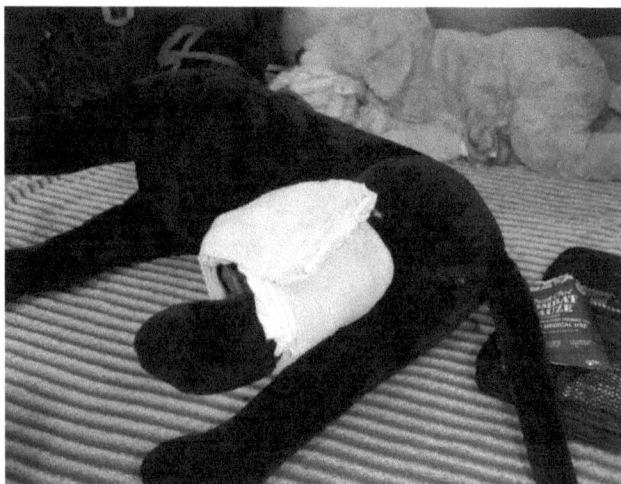

Tourniquets

The benefit of tourniquet use in human patients with massive hemorrhage has been proven and is now the standard of care for humans, but does present some issues with effectiveness in canines.

I have left the human tourniquet section in this book so you can have information to not only save your pet, but humans as well.

Tourniquets for Pets

While tourniquets are truly life-saving in both people and pets there are some draw backs when using them on a dog.

This is how I think of it - A human has a round leg and arm and a tourniquet will fit securely around the extremity if properly applied.

However, a dog has thin and narrow legs which may cause a human tourniquet, like the CAT or SOFTT-W, to loosen and slip down.

There is now a tourniquet specifically designed for dogs made by TacMed Solutions. I'll go over it more in-depth shortly.

Other tourniquets that may work on a dog are the SWAT-T and RAT. I'll go over these shortly as well.

While the SWAT-T and RAT can also be used to stop bleeding in humans the TacMed Solutions K9 Tourniquet is for animal use only.

According to the K9 Tactical Combat Casualty Care Guidelines, human designed tourniquets may not be effective or warranted in a K9 extremity bleed. Wound packing may in fact be the better option. I will cover tourniquets so you have all the knowledge you need to make a decision.

Tourniquet Do's & Don'ts

Remember Tourniquets are for extremities ONLY

1. Place the tourniquet above the affected joint. Never over top of a joint! (Joints in the arm are the wrist, elbow, shoulder. Joints in the leg are ankle, knee, and hip.)

2. High & Tight! Apply the tourniquet as high on the limb as possible and above the wound. Never place the tourniquet directly over the wound or on a joint!

3. Tighten until bleeding stops and there is no distal pulse (the pulse in the farthest point on the extremity).

4. Tell EMS or the Emergency Vet/ hospital there is a tourniquet on the victim you are with.

Types of Tourniquets

In the current guidelines for K9 TCCC if a tourniquet is to be used on a canine for massive bleeding consider the SWAT-T.

Using a Swat T tourniquet step by step

A SWAT-T tourniquet can be effective when used on a dog.

Because it is so wide and it must be placed above the wound and not over it, this can be a draw back when using it on a dog.

On the next few pages, you will see a step-by-step application of a SWAT-T on a human leg and a plush dog leg.

SWT: Stretch, Wrap and Tuck Tourniquet.

Human Images source: Marc Barry - Officer Survival Solutions.

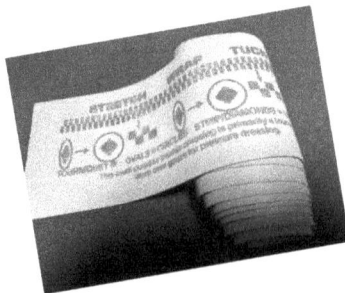

Deploy SWAT-T Tourniquet and Stretch it tight. Wrap it above the wound and as high on the limb as possible – not over a joint.

Human

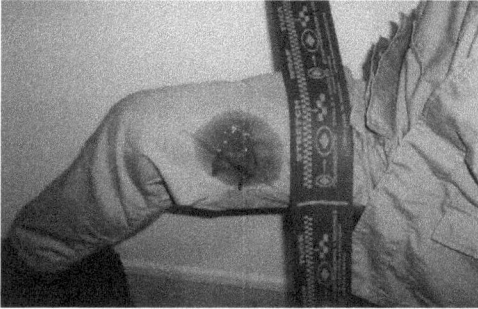

Pet

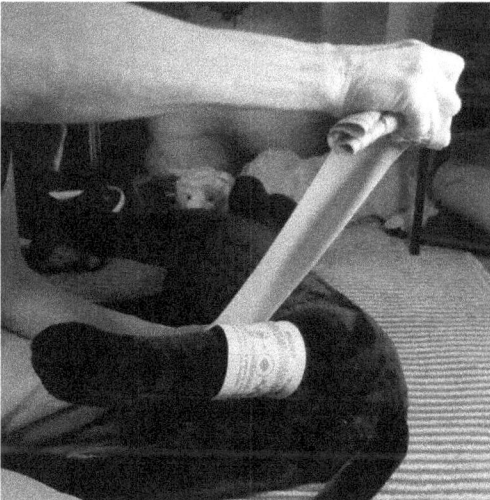

Continue the wrapping process to ensure tightness with each wrap.

Human

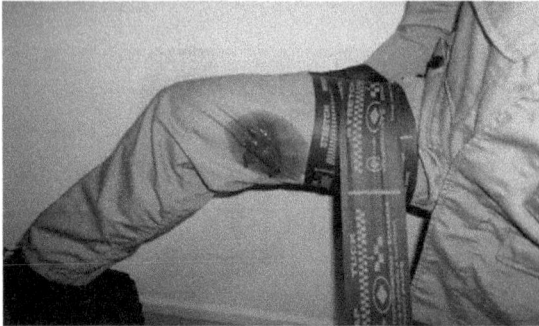

Pet

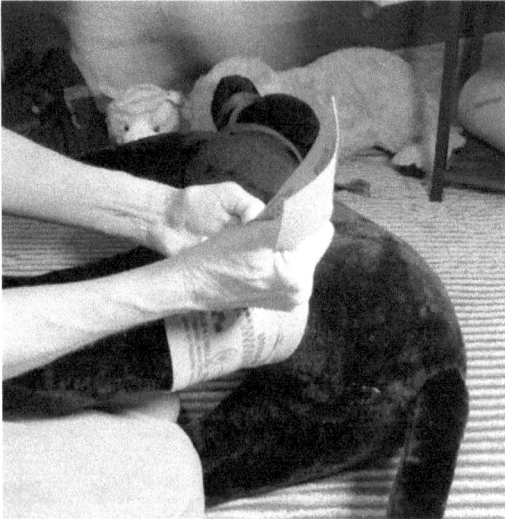

As you come to the last few inches, tuck the end of the tourniquet inside the wrap to secure it.

Human

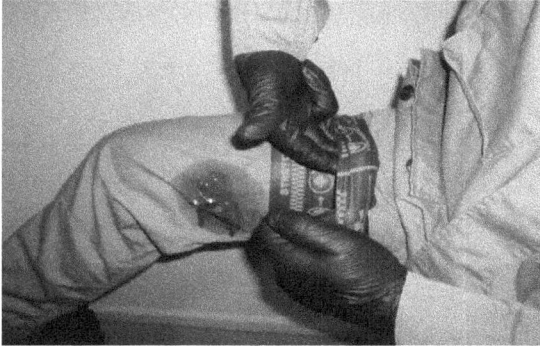

Pet

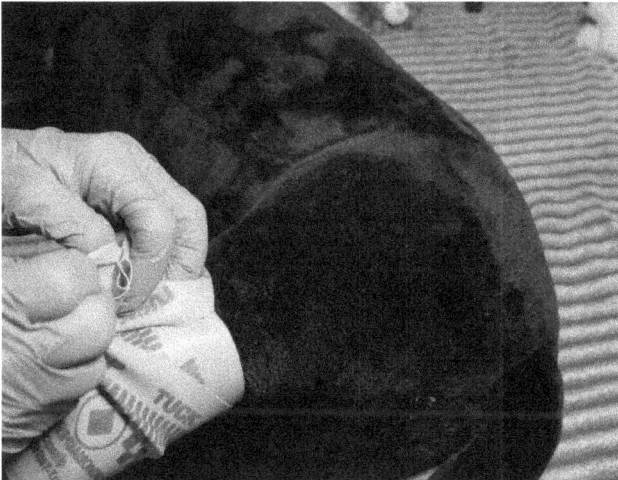

Properly applied -Human

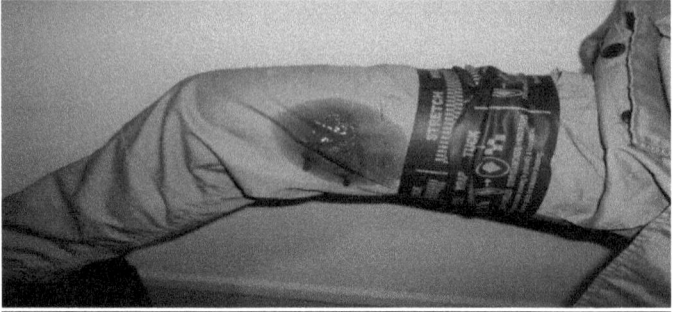

Properly applied - Pet

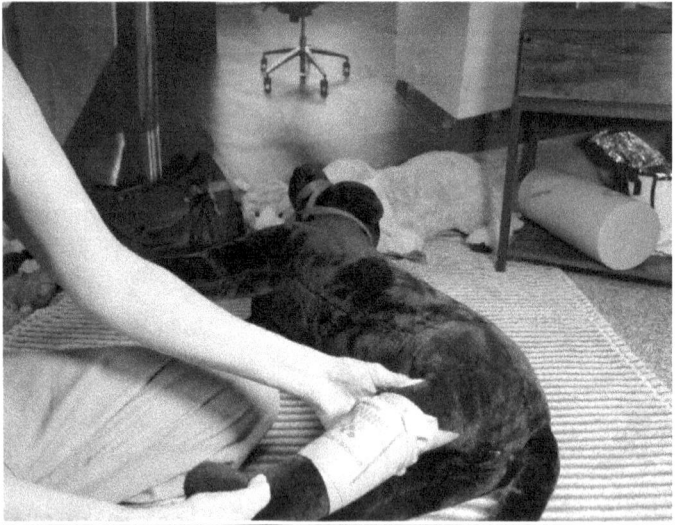

TACMED K9 Tourniquet

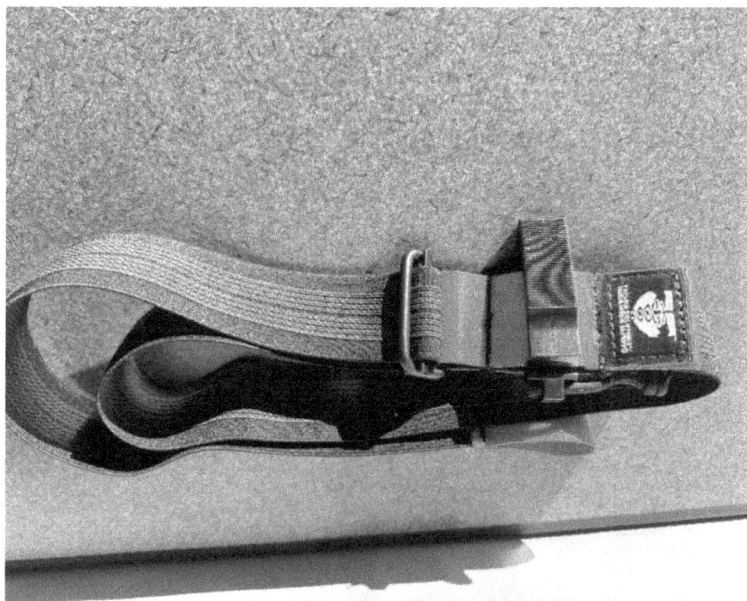

The TacMed K9 Tourniquet is designed specifically for dogs.

This K9 tourniquet is designed to mold to the dog's leg and, when applied high on the dog's leg, prevents it from slipping down.

This tourniquet is NOT designed for use on humans!

Steps to apply a TacMed K9 Tourniquet
1. Position the TQ over the limb and as high as possible.

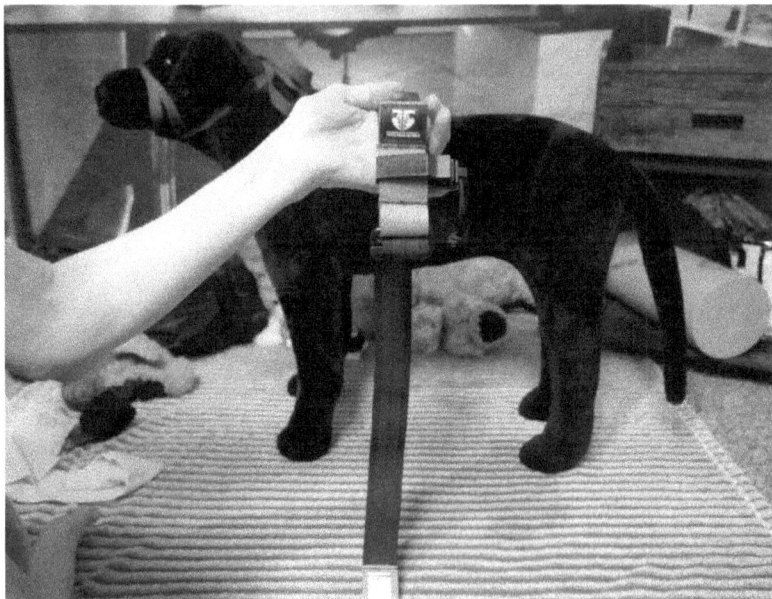

2. Tighten the TQ using the thumb anchor (a black ring - TacMed written on it) and pulling on the strap. Make it as tight around the limb as possible.

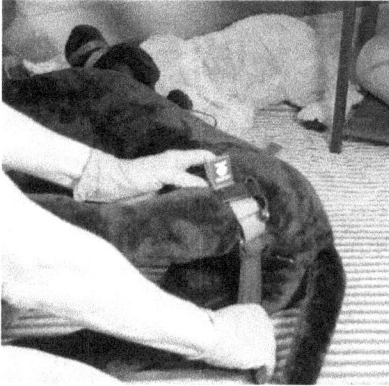

3. Tightly stretch and wrap the black webbing band above the initial placed part of the TQ. Wrap it around the limb until all bleeding stops. This black webbing placed above the initial site of the TQ will then anchor it and prevent slippage.

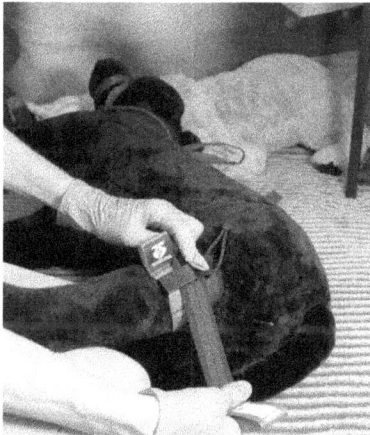

4.. Put the tail of the webbing band into the clip and press down, locking it in place.

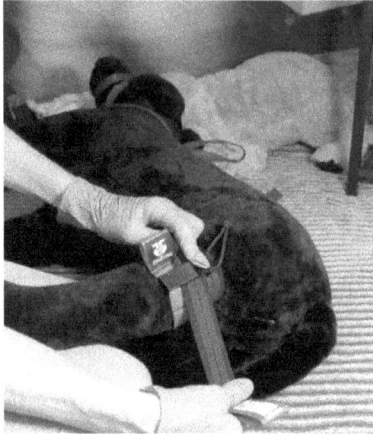

5. Reassess that all bleeding has stopped.

You can watch a video on how to apply this tourniquet on our website – www.traintorespond.com or on the TacMed YouTube channel.
I highly recommend watching the video as it will visually help cement the steps of application.

RAT - Rapid Application Tourniquet

The RAT TQ may be another option for stopping bleeding in an animal or person.

Rats Medical defines the RAT as: R.A.T. – *Rapid Application Tourniquet* – A solid vulcanized rubber core with a nylon sheath combined with a unique locking mechanism make this a simple and incredibly fast tourniquet to apply to self or others. The RAT's hallmark is "use under stress". The RAT TQ can be applied to a pet's leg and may be effective in stopping bleeding.

Image courtesy of Rats Medical

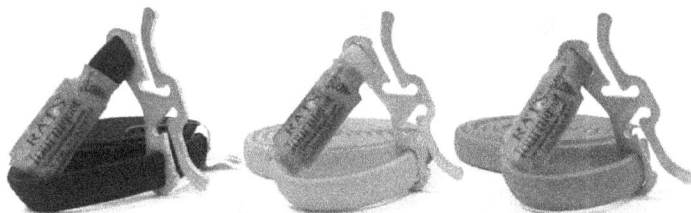

U.S. PAT. NO. 9,168,044

Using a RAT

Hold the metal cleat.
Below the cleat you will see a small loop
(called the three fingered loop).

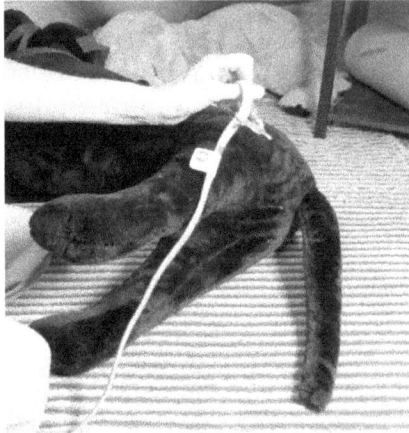

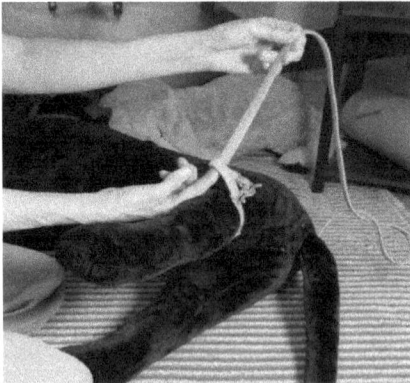

Thread the end of the tourniquet through the three
fingered loop.

(Do not widen the loop to place the limb through it).

Move the big loop you have created over the limb and start wrapping the band as tightly as possible around the limb.

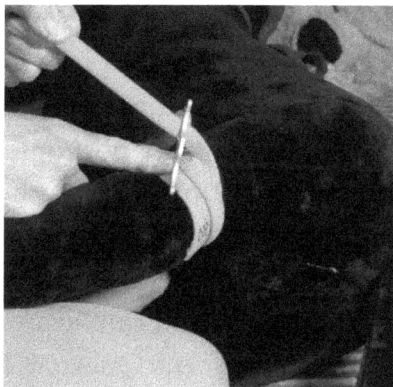

The band should NOT be wrapped on top of itself, but right next to itself around the extremity.

When the bleeding has stopped you then put the band of the RAT into the end of the cleat to secure it in place.

CAT - Combat Application Tourniquet

A CAT is a truly effective tool that, when used correctly, stops bleeding in **human extremities**.

According to the K9TCCC a tourniquet with a windlass such as the CAT or SOFTT-W are designed for humans and tend to slip down the much narrower leg of an animal. They also may not conform to the shape of an animal's leg. However, these are truly lifesaving in humans and I would be remiss not to include this for the human reading this manual.

The CAT is patented and can be applied using one hand. It is, as I call it – The Queen & King of Tourniquets for people.

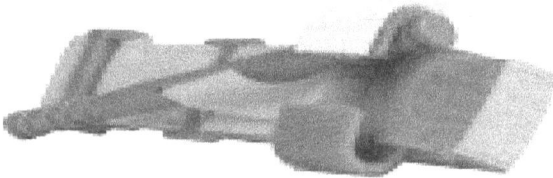

You can learn the steps for use on a human below.

1. Apply the CAT around and as high on the limb as possible Place it above the wound. Never place the tourniquet over top of the wound or on a joint!

2. The first pull on the constricting band is most important. Make the band as tight as possible around the limb.

3. Turn the windlass until bleeding stops and there is no distal pulse. Distal pulse is the pulse farthest in the extremity – wrist, foot.
4. Tuck the windlass in the windlass clip and pull the white band over top of it.
5. Write the time of application on the white band.
6. Keep reassessing the victim and tighten or apply a second tourniquet if bleeding has not stopped.

To learn more, go to North American Rescue https://www.narescue.com/

Image courtesy of North American Rescue

RECAP of Tourniquet Do's & Don'ts

Remember Tourniquets are for extremities ONLY

1. Place the tourniquet above the affected joint. Never over top of a joint!

2. High & Tight! Apply the tourniquet as high on the limb as possible and above the wound. Never over top of the wound or over a joint!

3. Tighten until bleeding stops and there is no distal pulse.

4. Tell EMS or the Emergency Vet / hospital there is a tourniquet on the victim you are with.

Training videos are also available on
The Train To Respond, LLC- YouTube channel.

<u>MArch</u> - **Airway**

Is the airway open and patent?
No!

Dog – open the dog's airway by lifting the head into alignment with the neck. This is a straight in-line position of the head and neck.

Pull the tongue out to look inside and make sure there is no obstruction. If you cannot clear the obstruction, transport to the vet immediately.

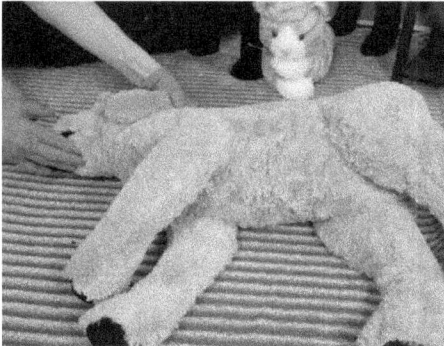

NOTE: Never practice rescue breathing or CPR on a live pet or animal!
MaRch - Respirations

Is the dog breathing?

No!

Immediately close the mouth and perform mouth to snout breathing.

You are blowing into the nose while keeping the mouth closed with your hands. Give enough air to make the chest rise, but do not over inflate the lungs.

Rescue breathing can vary depending on the size of the animal.

General guidelines are to give a breath every 3 – 6 seconds.

Puppies, cats, very small dog guidelines are one breath every 3 seconds.

Larger breed guidelines are one breath every 6 seconds.

This mirrors human pediatric and adult CPR guidelines.

MarCh – Circulation & chest injuries

Canine CPR Guidelines
NEVER PRACTICE ON A LIVE DOG!!
This will cause injury and harm to your pet!!!

Check for unresponsiveness – approach from the side or back calling their name & making noise.

Unresponsive – Yes!

Check for breathing – open the airway by aligning the pet's head/neck(think head tilt chin lift in human CPR) – look, listen and feel for breathing - not breathing – pull out tongue slightly – close mouth and seal your mouth over the dog's nose and blow into the dog's nose giving two breaths.

Breaths goes in – Yes - Check for pulse on the animals back leg (femoral artery)– no pulse – start chest compressions.

A good idea is to practice locating the pulse on your dog so that in the event you need to determine life or death you know exactly where to place your fingers.

NO PULSE – Begin chest compressions.

Hand Placement How you position your dog will depend on their breed, size and shape.

<u>Recommended dog and hand positions</u>

Medium - Large dog – Place dog on their side. Compress with hands placed directly behind dog's front leg/armpit. This is the area closest to the dog's heart.

Puppy – small dog – Perform CPR by cupping your hand. One hand underneath dog and other hand over chest. Use top hand to compress.

Barrel Chested Dog – Place on back and compress in center of dog's chest. Place your hands in the center of the dog's chest much like human CPR.

Do 30 compressions Push down on the chest one third of the way and then give **2 breaths**.

Do CPR for 2 minutes (5 times of 30-2) and then recheck for pulse and breathing.

Compress at a Rate of 100-120 per minute and allow full chest recoil (keep hands on chest) Think of the song – Staying Alive.

Rescue breathing –Dog has a pulse, but is not breathing. Initiate mouth to snout breaths- general guidelines are to **give one breath approximately every 3 seconds for small**

animals and one breath approximately every 6 seconds for larger animals.

I strongly suggest you take an in-person Pet CPR class. In our live training classes, we do hands on practice assessing, providing emergency care and CPR & Choking. Contact us at traintorespond.com

I can also highly recommend a class I attended. It was taught by the owner of Paws N Claws 911, Tom Rinelli.

He offers in-person training and you can find his schedule of classes at www.pawsnclaws911.com.

Never practice CPR or rescue breathing on a live animal as this could cause great harm.

Take a K9 or Pet First Aid class and get real hands-on practice.

You can also find online training on our website at traintorespond.com

Chest injuries

If your pet suffers a penetrating injury to the chest and has an open/sucking chest wound, they require immediate treatment.

Your main goal is to cover the open hole and assess for an exit wound and cover that as well.

Think of it this way - Air goes in by path of least resistance – the mouth and nose. However, if there is a hole or holes in the chest/back/belly, air will go in there as well.

As air begins to accumulate in the chest cavity it presses on the lungs and heart and can cause death.

By covering the hole or holes with an air-tight (occlusive dressing) you prevent extra air from entering the cavity.

<u>Steps to treat an open / sucking chest wound:</u>

Cover the hole or holes with your gloved hand and then replace with an occlusive dressing.

Pets present an issue with how well the seal will work if there is a lot of hair.

You may need to use a razor or clippers to shave hair around the wound and allow the occlusive dressing to stick on the skin.

The occlusive seal must be against the skin to truly work. They make commercial chest seals such as the Hyfin.

If you do not have a commercial seal then improvise with anything that is air-tight. Plastic bag, glove, etc.... Tape down all four sides of whatever you use.

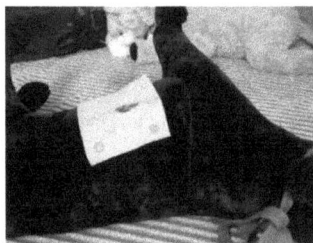

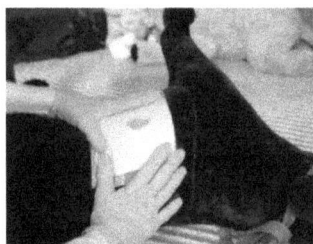

Hyfin Chest Seal

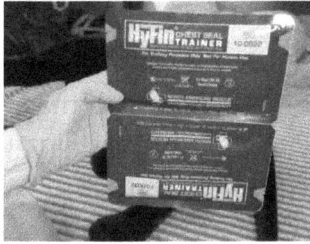

Open pack and peel off Hyfin chest seal

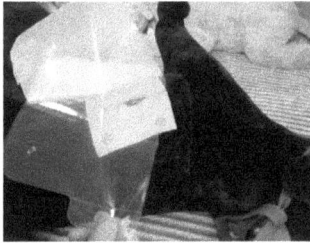

Place Hyfin over the wound & press glue side down

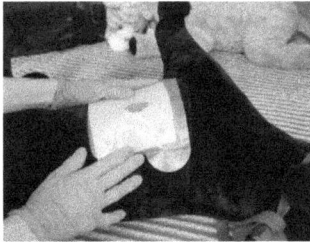

You must now watch the animal closely to see if they are developing a condition called a tension pneumothorax.

Watch for increasingly severe respiratory distress agitation, rapid breathing, absent breath sounds on one side of their chest, shock (weak pulses, pale gums)

If these symptoms present, then you will do what we call "burping the seal." Burping the seal is to simply lift up one side, allow the animal to exhale, and reseal it. This allows air to escape. You may do this multiple times on the way to the vet. At the vet they will insert a needle to decompress the chest and allow air to escape.

This requires immediate transportation to an emergency vet!

Marc**H** – **Hypothermia**

Keeping an injured pet warm is vital. Keeping a pet with massive blood loss warm, is lifesaving.

As with people, if you allow your traumatically injured pet to become cold/hypothermic, they can die.

Hypothermia is a true killer! When a person or pet's body temperature drops and they become hypothermic (cold) their body stops being able to form clots and stop bleeding.

There is something we call in emergency medicine The Deadly Triad of Trauma. I don't want to go in-depth in this process, but the basics are these three issues

Hypothermia - cold

Coagulopathy – body can't form clots

Acidosis – body becomes acidotic and cannot function.

The one thing we can help with, as rescuers, at the point of injury is keeping the pet warm.

Hypothermia prevention and treatment: Place blankets below them and over them, use a sleeping bag or survival blanket. Use whatever will retain heat and help them stay warm.

Turn on the heat. Remove any wet or blood-soaked outerwear or booties.

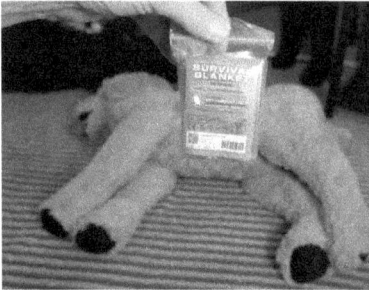

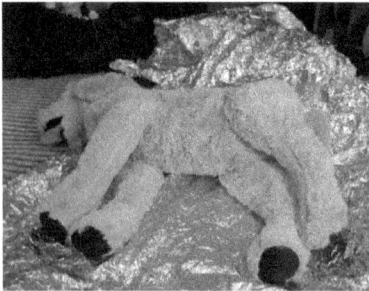

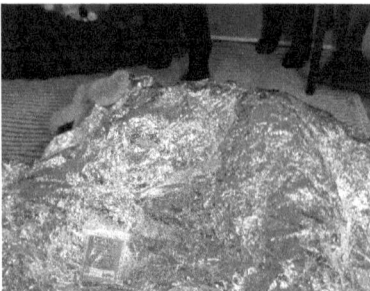

Positioning your injured Canine

Conscious animals – allow them to stay in a position of comfort, unless contraindicated by their condition.

Unconscious – place them in the **recovery position.**

1. Open their airway.

2. Place on right side to reduce pressure on the heart.

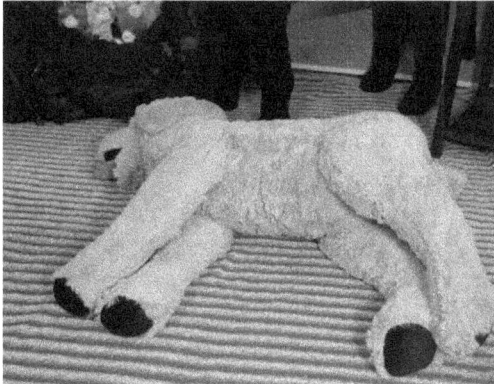

T – Transport

It is vital you transport your pet to the emergency vet safely.

Stay calm. Animals pick up on our fears and this can increase their anxiety and heart rate.

Put the address in your GPS so you do not have to stress over directions.

Put your pet in a carrier, if feasible.

If your pet is larger, you will need a way to get them to your vehicle.

There are disposable litters we use on rescue task forces that you can purchase and are fairly inexpensive.

Blanket drags are also an option if you are unable to physically carry your pet.

If you can find another person to ride with you, that is the best way to go. One person can monitor and continue treatment while the other can drive.

Many times, I have seen Law Enforcement step up and assist injured animals and their pet parents. Know your non-emergency police number if you require assistance.

By following SMART and MARCH you can help your dog get the best outcome possible.

SMART

Scene safety, Muzzle, Assess, Rapidly Treat, Transport.

MARCH

Massive bleeding control, Airway, Respirations, Circulation, Hypothermia

Module Six
Special Circumstances

Impaled objects

Perform a rapid assessment to find life threatening injuries or problems.

1. Treat life threatening problems or injuries immediately.

2. Leave impaled object in and stabilize it. You can use gauze rolls on each side of the object and then wrap around them with gauze. Whatever works, the goal is to leave the object in and get to the emergency vet asap!

**The reason we leave impaled objects in is that the object itself may be what is sealing off the bleeding artery. To remove it would cause massive bleeding as well as further injury to organs.

3. If the object is large, such as a fence post, it may require extrication/cutting so the animal can be transported, object in place, to the vet.

4. Treat major bleeding.

Impaled object treatment

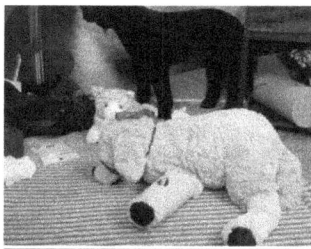

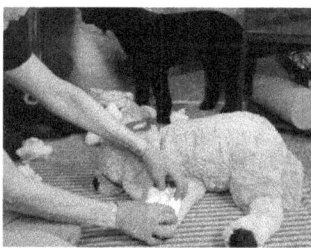

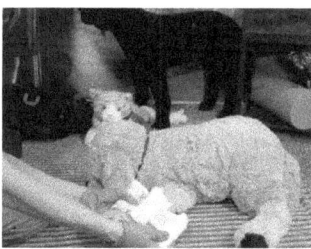

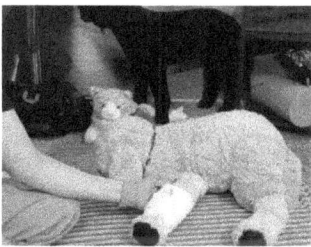

Fractures

If your dog suffers a fracture of an extremity or their tail you may need to splint it for transportation to the emergency vet.

There are many things you can use as a splint. It will depend on the size of the animal as to what you use for splint.

Here are some items to consider: a pillow, cardboard, a rigid stick, a magazine, tongue depressors. You get the idea. Something that is rigid, the right size and weight for your pet and one that you will be able to secure.

When splinting an injured animal or person here are steps to follow:

1. If it is an open fracture (the bone is sticking out or exposed) – do not push it back in!

2. You may put a loose, sterile dressing over the bone.

3. Apply the splint and make sure it is long enough to immobilize above and below the break and the joints above and below the break.

4. Pad any voids between the splint and the animal's leg.

5. Do not tie so tightly that you cut off blood supply.

The goal of a splint is to prevent movement of the fractured extremity and to help reduce pain, especially during transport to the vet.

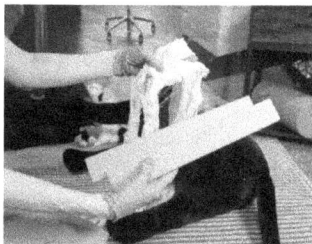

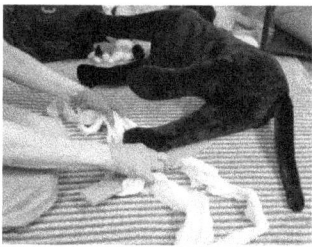

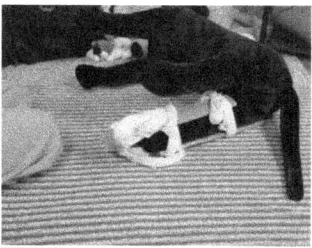

Suspected Spinal Injury

If you suspect your pet has suffered an injury to their spine or back, it is vital that you move them as little as possible.

Immobilize them in the position found and on a rigid object or board.

You will need help to slide the injured animal, as a unit, onto the board.

Hold stabilization of the pet to prevent movement and reassure them with a calm voice.

Transport to an emergency vet.

Tail Injuries

Tails, believe it or not, are part of a dog's spine. There are arteries and veins running though their tails and, if an artery is injured, massive bleeding can occur.

If a pet gets a severe tail injury, this can impact their spine, so be alert if they lose bowel or bladder control. This can signify a spinal cord injury and not just a simple tail issue.

For minor tail wounds – assess the injury, flush it for debris, apply first aid ointment and dress and bandage using gauze pads and gauze wrap.

Internal Bleeding

It can be difficult to determine internal bleeding. If your pet has suffered blunt force trauma there may be no obvious injury.

In people, we look for bruising and this is not easy to see in a pet due to their fur.

If there is history of any type of blunt trauma and your pet isn't acting right or appears in pain, be on high alert.

Check their vital signs. Is their heart rate really fast? Check their gums – do they appear pale? Is your pet lethargic? Are they weak?

These can all be signs your pet may have internal bleeding and is going into shock.

Transport immediately to the emergency vet for evaluation.

Bite Wounds

Sadly, bite wounds are something I am very familiar with. My two sweet greyhounds were out for a walk with their pet sitter one day while I was at work. As they were walking by a house with an invisible fence, a chocolate lab suddenly charged them (the invisible fence did not work!) and started attacking both my girls.

Greyhounds are the sweetest beings and are not prepared for something like this. They were bitten and ripped to shreds in multiple places on their bodies.

Thankfully, my amazing pet sitter was able to scream for help and the dog's owners came out and got the dog off my two girls.

My pet sitter notified me about what had happened and that she was transporting them to the emergency vet. I immediately called my supervisors and told them I was leaving and they needed to get a paramedic in to replace me. I headed to the vet and found, once there, both my girls were in surgery.

I am grateful to the expertise of the vets as they saved both girls. They were in the hospital for a few days and then came home, where I basically set up an intensive care unit.

They required medications every four hours, bandage changes and help doing anything and everything.

I was out of work for two weeks (it was just me and I had no one to help me) and when I came back I was summoned down to the office. It was the one and only time in my entire career as a paramedic I was given a written warning.

I know in some people's hearts, animals aren't family. But to me, they were my fur-daughters, and I would do anything for them. I'd do it again in a heartbeat, no matter what the cost.

If your pet has a bite wound or wounds, they may be deeper than they look. You also have no idea if there are internal injuries that you can't see. You also need to know the rabies vaccination status of the animal that bit your pet.

For a bite wound – assess, clean flush, control bleeding and transport to the emergency vet. Your pet may need antibiotics and pain meds, like my girls did.

My sweet girl, Queen of the Nights, well into her healing stage after the dog attack.

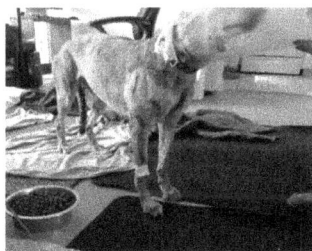

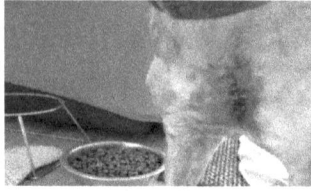

My sweet girl, KD Kelsey, with staples still in her wounds, but beginning to heal and feeling a bit better.

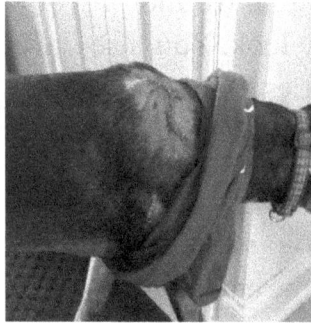

Thankfully my greyhounds were used to wearing shirts, and all kinds of things, because they need to stay warm. So, I kept both girls in tee shirts and this helped cover their wounds.

Foot Injuries

Another issue I became very well versed in with my greyhounds was paw, nail and foot injuries.

I can't count the number of times they came in from playing together outside with a trail of blood following. I'd stop and have to examine each of them to see who hurt their foot.

Most of the time it was a cut to the paw or pad, but one time Miss KD Kelsey ripped off her toenail. Talk about bleeding!

If your pet suffers a paw or foot wound treat it as you would any wound.

Assess – clean, flush, and stop the bleeding.

I got very good at dressing the wounds with a gauze pad, ace bandage or roller gauze and then using this amazing bootie created by Ilaria Borghese of Thera Paw!

My two girls and I would volunteer at an animal wellness event and one of the companies there was Thera Paw. Miss Queen of the Nights had a racing injury and only had three toes. One had been amputated and she had difficulty balancing sometimes.

Ilaria saw her and handcrafted the boot you see below for her to wear when she had difficulty. I still have the boot and hope, when I can adopt or foster more greyhounds, it will once again come in handy.

When either of my girls had paw injuries I would dress and bandage the foot and then apply the bootie.

Let me tell you, I could let them go out and play and the bootie stayed on. It rarely ever came off and it helped my greys lead as normal a life as they could when a paw or foot was injured. You can check out Thera Paw and all their pet products at www.therapaw.com. I highly recommend them!

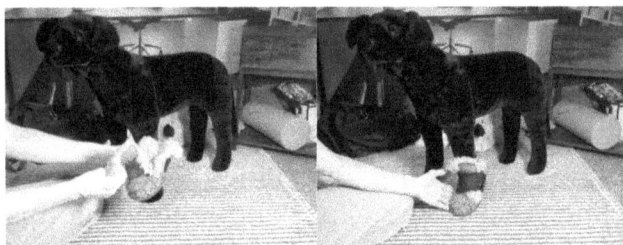

I don't know about you, but I absolutely dreaded clipping my dog's nails! It is hard to judge where the quick (blood vessel) is in dark colored nails. If you clip the quick it will start to bleed and cause pain to your pet!

Don't panic. Most nail bleeds can be stopped by applying direct pressure to the quick. I also used to use styptic powder. This is a medication / powder that you can apply to the quick and it helps stop bleeding.

Styptic powder is not to be used for major bleeding and certainly not for arterial bleeds. That would be where Quick Clot or Celox comes in. However, it works great for minor nail bleeds. It comes under a variety of names and you can find it online or at your pet store.

Shock

The definition of shock is inadequate tissue perfusion. Basically, it means that the tissues and organs are not getting enough blood and oxygen to function properly.

Shock can happen with many injuries and illnesses. This is why it is important to do your assessment.

Are their gums pale or cyanotic? Yes = shock = lack of oxygen.

Is their heart rate really rapid? Yes = may be shock or a cardiac issue.

Is your pet acting lethargic and weak? Yes = may be shock.

If your pet is bleeding – stop the bleeding and keep them warm.

Transport any animal that has signs and symptoms of shock to the emergency vet for evaluation!

<u>BLOAT – A dire emergency</u>

I remember it being a dark night and my yellow lab, Barky Bear, wasn't acting right. My paramedic Spidey senses were on high alert. He was lethargic, and not his happy self.

Now, these things never seem to happen during the day and if you are a pet parent, I am sure you know this.

I stayed up with him and he started to have dry heaves and was keeping his head down and his back bunched up.

I decided to take him to the twenty-four-hour veterinary hospital that was closest to me. This would be the same twenty-four-hour veterinary hospital that years later saved my greyhounds. A different time and different doctors!

I arrived with Barky around midnight and entered the vet. He was clearly getting worse. They kept me waiting because there was a cat that the vet was seeing.

Finally, they brought us into a room and this little blonde vet walked in

The vet pushed on his belly, did a cursory exam and clearly didn't think it was anything major. At this point Barky Bear begins vomiting and has thick ropey saliva drooling out of his mouth.

She then leaves the room and does not call in a vet tech or order any testing.

A couple minutes later I went out to the desk. I knew Barky was in bad shape and I wanted to know where the vet went. The person at the desk said results were back for the cat and she was looking at them.

I asked if the cat was stable? The person at the desk told me that the cat was stable and they had just been worried it has been poisoned by something.

I said, "well, something is really wrong with my dog and I need the vet back in the room now." Five minutes later – no vet. I left the room with Barky and told them I was leaving.

I remember driving back home. I had a pickup with one of those rear windows and Barky would always stick his head out and enjoy the ride. I was thinking am I wrong? Am I making too big a deal out of this? The vet didn't think anything was seriously wrong.

I was about to head home when I looked back towards Barky. His head was down. He wasn't looking out the window and appeared in pain.

I knew where another twenty-four-hour vet was and after looking at him I changed course and headed directly there. It was called Alliance Animal Hospital in Roxbury, NJ. It was further away, but I am so glad I listened to my gut and trusted my assessment and took him there.

We arrived and we walked in. Dr. Hamilton came in immediately to exam him. She knew right away something was wrong and they took him in the back. It was around two in the morning and she told me to go home and she would call me once she knew more.

I didn't want to go, but she was right. Barky was in their hands now. I went home, didn't sleep, and waited by the phone. Finally in the morning hours, Dr. Hamilton called.

She told me that he had Bloat. His spleen had torsioned (twisted) and cut off all blood flow to his intestines and organs. She operated and said that when she opened him up, everything was blue (cyanotic – no oxygen) and she thought they would have to put him down.

Miraculously, when she untwisted the spleen, blood flow restored and things began to pink up! My prayers had been answered.

Barky was in intensive care there for a number of days, so I would go down and visit him every day.

Now you can imagine the cost! I was grateful I was able to take out a credit card, especially for vet emergencies and pay it off over time.

Barky Bear and I got to enjoy many more years of walks and fun and love. It was well worth every penny.

I am forever grateful to you Dr. Hamilton and the staff of the now closed Alliance Animal Hospital.

Imagine, I know I do, if I had seconded guessed my gut and driven home that night! If I had decided that little blonde vet was on the right track and nothing serious was wrong. Imagine my guilt and the horrific and painful death my yellow lab would have suffered.

If I can impress anything on you, it is to trust your gut. Trust what you know and what you feel. It has helped me not only with my animals, but in my career as a paramedic. I always say "Your gut will never steer you wrong."

Bloat is life threatening!! I was blessed that Barky hung in there for hours. Sometime Bloat kills very quickly.

Bloat has a very high mortality rate.

When an animal has bloat, GDV or gastric distention occurs. The stomach fills up and puts pressure on organs, arteries, veins and, in Barky's case, his spleen.

This pressure causes volvulus or twisting of the stomach or organ and this cuts off blood flow.

Bloat mainly occurs in large dogs with deep and narrow chests. If any of these symptoms or signs happen to your animal, no matter their size, get them to the vet.

Signs & symptoms of Bloat

Pacing

Anxiety

Dry vomit

Drooling – thick, rope-like – gooey saliva (Barky had this)

Head down

Back bunched

Swelling near rib cage

Whimpering

Pain

If these symptoms or some of these symptoms occur then please take your pet to the vet for evaluation.

What might cause Bloat?

After experiencing bloat with Barky, I started researching what could have caused this.

Here are some things I found out and it did change how I feed and when I fed or let my dogs drink water after exercise

Possible causes of Bloat:

Vigorous exercise after a meal

Large meal

Gulping food

Gulping large amounts of water after a meal or exercise

I also believe, personally, that the rawhide bones I'd been giving Barky may have had something to do with the bloat.

I stopped using rawhide after the bloat episode.

This is my experience with Bloat and I pray you never have to have a similar one.

Heat Emergencies

Heat Emergencies

Heat can be deadly emergencies for K9's

Dogs lose heat through panting!

They may sweat a small bit through the pads of their feet.

With their fur and inability to sweat heat can cause death for a K9.

Treatment for heat stroke & heat emergencies!

Remove them from the heat source – sun – vehicle etc.. Move them to a cool area.

If they are a K9 officer wearing a vest – remove it and their collar.

Apply a slip leash.

Let them lay on their side and gradually drink water. NO GULPING!

Pat them lightly with wet towels against the fur – can help them to evaporate heat.

Note: Saturated wet fur can hold in heat. When patting them with wet towels push the hair in opposite direction. This will open up their coat.

Module Seven

Preparing to give report to the Emergency Vet

It is good to know the information the emergency vet and team will need to know upon their arrival.

The questions asked are in the quest to get a complete and detailed picture of your pet's condition.

A clear picture of what is wrong will assist the emergency responders in their treatment and decision making for your fur-baby.

A good way to remember the basic information emergency vets or even human first responders will need is the acronym is the word - SAMPLE

Try to have the following pertinent information written down, to give to the emergency responders when they arrive.

1. Pets name.

2. Pet's age or date of birth.

Use the acronym – SAMPLE

S – Signs and Symptoms your pet is having or has had before arriving at the vet.

A - Allergies your pet has.

M - Medications your pet is taking.

P - Pertinent medical history of your pet.

L - Last oral intake. This is very important if your pet is facing immediate surgery for their condition.

E - Events leading up to the current illness or injury. What happened before the emergency responders arrived?

Trauma Kits

There are many different types of trauma kits specifically designed for treating severe arterial bleeding and gunshot/stabbing injuries. Consider these items when putting together a trauma kit.

1. Medical Gloves

2. Tourniquet (Swat T, TacMed, Rat, (CAT - human use.)

3. Hemostatic Gauze (Celox or Quick Clot)

4. Pressure Bandage

5. Hyfin Chest Vented Seals - Two

6. Muzzle

7. Blanket

8. Leash

9. Gauze pads & roller gauze

10. First Aid ointment

11. Sterile water to flush debris

Each piece of equipment is vitally important in treating a severely injured pet.

If you get a chance to attend one of our in-person K9 Tactical First Aid or Pet First Aid for Dogs & Cats training classes, we will go over, in depth, how to utilize each piece of equipment.

Keeping a first aid kit on hand is a good idea. I keep one in my car and carry smaller ones in my purse and backpack.

It is important to cover any open cuts and bleeding wounds on yourself before providing care.

This is why you should have non latex medical gloves with you at all times.

I keep medical glove in my purse, car, and take them any place I go where I may have to help someone.

Here are the companies I personally purchase my emergency equipment and training equipment from.

It is vital you purchase from a reputable company as there have been fake tourniquets and equipment put out there by not so reputable companies.

I recommend the following and do not receive any compensation for doing so. They are truly the ones I have purchased from and had a great experience with.

My trusted companies:

1. North American Rescue
2. TacMed Solutions
3 Rescue Essentials
4. Ready Man

I have also purchased equipment from amazon.com, but please make sure you know the listed company is the genuine thing before you purchase.

Conclusion

Thank you for investing in yourself, your family, friends, co-workers and the future of our world.

Together we can make a difference and empower ourselves to help our injured pets or other animals.

At Train To Respond, LLC we provide training for Active Threat / Shooting Response, Bleed Control Specialist training for Pets and People and Rescue Task Force Training.

In-person with hands on training and practice is the preferred method, however, we do also offer online training if you can't make an in-person class. Our trainings are available at www.traintorespond.com.

For further information or to schedule training for your company or group please email us at: traintorespond@gmail.com

Our training is available for families, communities, businesses, groups, organizations, entertainment venues, places of worship, gun ranges & clubs and schools.

Email us today at traintorespond@gmail.com or visit us at www.traintorespond.com

Resources

Our bleeding control training follows the recommendations of the TCCC - Tactical Combat Casualty Care and TECC - Tactical Emergency Casualty Care and K9 TCCC.

Works cited

1. Canine – Tactical Combat Casualty Care Guideline

2. In-person Training from Paws N Claws 911 - Tom Rinelli.

3. National Safety Council

Notes

www.ingramcontent.com/pod-product-compliance
Lightning Source LLC
Chambersburg PA
CBHW060511280326
41933CB00014B/2924